Katerine Sacoto Quinteros

Drug addiction in adolescents

Katerine Sacoto Quinteros

Drug addiction in adolescents

Drug addiction in adolescents treated at the duran hospital in the years 2013-2015

ScienciaScripts

Imprint
Any brand names and product names mentioned in this book are subject to trademark, brand or patent protection and are trademarks or registered trademarks of their respective holders. The use of brand names, product names, common names, trade names, product descriptions etc. even without a particular marking in this work is in no way to be construed to mean that such names may be regarded as unrestricted in respect of trademark and brand protection legislation and could thus be used by anyone.

Cover image: www.ingimage.com

This book is a translation from the original published under ISBN 978-620-3-03721-0.

Publisher:
Sciencia Scripts
is a trademark of
International Book Market Service Ltd., member of OmniScriptum Publishing Group
17 Meldrum Street, Beau Bassin 71504, Mauritius
Printed at: see last page
ISBN: 978-620-3-37876-4

DEDICATION

I dedicate this thesis to God and my family. To God because He has been with me every step I take, taking care of me and giving me strength to move forward in this long journey; To my family, my husband, my daughters, my brothers, but especially to my parents who throughout my life have become the foundation of my life and the strength that drives me to move forward in the goals I have set, being my support at all times, depositing their full confidence in every challenge I faced without doubting my ability and spirit of improvement.

Katerine Sacoto Quinteros

ACKNOWLEDGMENTS

This research work was carried out under the supervision of Dr. Patricia Párraga Pazmiño of the Hospital Básico de Duran, to whom I would like to express my sincere gratitude for making this study possible. I would like to thank her for her patience, time and dedication to make this study a success.

To God, for giving me the faith and strength to believe in my dreams and giving me the opportunity to continue to live in order to achieve them despite all the obstacles I have had on this long road.

To my parents, Nube and Eduardo for being the greatest and unconditional support during my college career, because without them I would not have achieved my goals and dreams. For being my example to follow, for teaching me to fight, to work and learn every day regardless of the circumstances and time.

To my siblings, Eduardo, Ronald and Doménica for trusting me, for always encouraging me to continue in all these long years, for helping me as well as my parents and Isabel in the care of my daughters Pamela and Angelline, to all of you I thank you for your words of encouragement that at some point in my life said and I always have them present in my mind, my heart and actions. You are all part of this dream, which today becomes a reality.

To my husband, Dario Parra, for all the patience and emotional support he has given me, as he gives me the confidence that I can achieve my dreams and that all this sacrifice is necessary for our future.To my great family, grandparents Nacho and Rosendo, uncles, aunts, cousins and cousins for never criticizing me and always supporting me and encouraging me to achieve this dream that is becoming a reality.To my colleagues and friends, who have passed through my life, for those who left and for those who stayed, thank you for putting up with me, I have memories of each one of them, good or bad, they always helped me to be a better person.

To my teachers, thank you because you shared with me your knowledge, your experiences, your life and contributed a lot in my career to now become a health professional, I will always carry you in my mind and in my heart.

Katerine Sacoto Quinteros

SUMMARY

Title: **"DROGADICCIONENADOLESCENTESATENDIDOEN.DURAN HOSPITAL IN THE YEARS 2014-2015".**

Author: SACOTO QUINTEROS KATERINE JANNETH

Objective: To determine the incidence of psychoactive substance use in adolescents and their predisposing factors for drug addiction through indirect observation to provide information to the service.

Methodology: A retrospective descriptive study was conducted, reviewing the medical records through the AS-400 system of all adolescent patients aged 10 to 19 years who consumed psychoactive substances attended in the emergency room of the Basic Hospital of Duran during the years 2014-2015. The medical records were collected by searching by ICD 10 code (diagnoses) and the data were organized using the Microsoft Excel statistical program.

Results: There was a predominance of males in relation to females, most cases were between 15 and 19 years of age, it was found that most of those affected were from the urban-marginal sector, mostly students and of low to medium social status, who had already had several previous episodes of consumption and had not sought help; it was determined that the most commonly used drug was cannabis. It was determined that part of the substance-consuming population had a history of psychiatric pathologies, most frequently depressive disorders, and frequently went to the emergency room for dependency syndrome.

Conclusions: Substance use continues to be a serious public health problem, there is little attention and resources allocated to its prevention and treatment therefore, it is important to strengthen continuing education plans and psychological support for adolescents and their families so functional and organic repercussions would be avoided in order to prevent fatal cases.

Keywords: Substances, Addiction, Dependence, Withdrawal Syndrome, Prevention.

ABSTRACT

Title: "DRUG ADDICTION IN ADOLESCENTS ATTENDED AT DURAN HOSPITAL IN THE YEARS 2014-2015".

Author: SACOTO QUINTEROS KATERINE JANNETH

Objective: To determine the incidence of use of psychoactive substances in adolescents and their predisposing factors for drug addiction through indirect observation to provide information to the service.

Methodology: A retrospective descriptive study was carried out. The clinical records were reviewed through the AS-400 system of all adolescents aged 10 to 19 years who used psychoactive substances treated during the emergency of the Duran Basic Hospital during the years 2014-2015. The collection of medical records was obtained by searching for CIE code 10 (diagnoses) and organizing the data using the statistical program Microsoft Excel.

Results: A predominance of males was shown in a relation to females, most cases occurred between 15 and 19 years, it was evidenced that those affected came from the urban-marginal sector, mostly from students of occupation and Of the low to middle social status, which had already presented several previous episodes of consumption and had not sought help; The most commonly used drug was cannabis. It was determined that a part of the population consumes of the substances presents antecedents of psychiatric pathologies, frequently of the majority of depressive disorders and frequently appeared to the emergency by dependency syndrome.

Conclusions: Consumption of chemical substances remains a public health problem, there is little attention and resources are devoted to its prevention and treatment, it is important to strengthen the plans for continuing education and psychological support for adolescents and their Family members so avoid functional and organic repercussions in order to avoid fatal cases.

Key Words: Substances, Addiction, Dependence, Abstinence Syndrome, Prevention.

INDEX

INTRODUCTION

Drug addiction is a disorder characterized by an uncontrollable desire to consume a certain substance, whether legal or not, to which a person has become accustomed after repeated use, called addiction. The problem of the consumption of psychoactive substances or commonly called drugs is no longer new in the world.

In itself, looking at the problem of drug use, we can conclude that it is a problem that affects the individual who is dependent on it and everyone because it is a transnational phenomenon that highlights the multifaceted nature of this scourge, its complex links with violence, criminal acts, its influence on the health and future of children and youth, and its negative impact on our country. (WHO, Drug Addiction, 2015) The use of psychoactive substances is an increasingly frequent factor and unfortunately the age of onset is much earlier than a decade ago, affecting not only this vulnerable group but also their families and society as a whole.

In general, a gratifying effect is sought, which may be the alteration of mental activity, attitudes or the degree of perception, however, their consumption often leads to mental imbalance even when they do not produce organic lesions.

It should also be emphasized that in order to talk about drug addiction in adolescents, we must think about the factors that lead adolescents to take refuge in drugs, which is why this study is detailed below, using statistics obtained from the HOSPITAL BASICO DURAN and various analyses that will be carried out for this assessment.

According to what will be studied below, it will be seen that the most vulnerable age for the beginning of drug use is currently between 12 and 16 years old, often starting with inhalants and then proceeding to the use of derivative drugs such as "hashish", a very harmful drug with disastrous side effects not only for the individual but also for the family and its environment. At this stage of life, the environments in which adolescents live are very influential: the family, which tends to lose control; the school where they spend most of their time, the groups of friends that are increasingly gaining prominence and the lack of permanent and adequate information on the subject.

The purpose of this degree work is to determine which are the most predisposing risk factors for adolescents to use different types of drugs.

The methods to be used in the elaboration of this work will be:

- Analysis of electronic medical records reviewed by prior acceptance of the statistics department of the HOSPITAL BASICO DURAN.
- Study of data obtained from national and international books or journals to perform this analysis.

CHAPTER I THE PROBLEM

PROBLEM STATEMENT

Currently in the canton of Duran many cases of drug addiction have been observed, which have even led adolescents to commit illegal acts, according to reports from the canton police and television interviews.

The most involved in this issue are low-income adolescents who often do not have the support of their parents and, feeling unprotected, take refuge in this vice without realizing how much it affects them.

According to the UN's annual report on drugs, an estimated 1 in 20 adults, or around 250 million people between the ages of 15 and 64, used at least one drug in 2014. Although considerable, that figure-roughly equivalent to the sum of the populations of France, Germany, Italy and the United Kingdom-does not appear to have increased over the past four years in proportion to the world's population. However, given that more than 29 million people who use drugs are estimated to suffer from drug-related disorders, and that 12 million of these people are injecting drug users, 14% of whom are living with HIV, the impact of drug use in terms of its health consequences remains devastating. (UNODC, 2016).

Reviewing a report carried out in the Duran canton. While on a side wall of the headquarters of the educational district of the Duran canton, murals painted by students from various schools encourage children to reject drug use, but, around the corner, in front of the Duran school, with relative discretion, a young man hands out packages to students who begin to leave the public establishment.

Mothers link the individual as one of the alleged drug dealers who daily are located outside this and other schools from 12:00 noon onwards. (Universo, 2015)

The sale and consumption of drugs among adolescents and young people, either outside schools or in the neighborhoods, is a constant problem in the railway city, the second most populated in Guayas with 235,769 inhabitants, according to the latest INEC census of 2010.

So far this year, 38,607 grams of drugs have been seized there, mainly cocaine hydrochloride. During 2014, 777,766 grams were seized, according to figures from the

Antinarcotics Police.

Ramiro Arequipa, captain of the Durán police district (with 379 uniformed officers), says that the distribution of narcotics outside schools is combated with operations and programs such as Vendedor Seguro and Escuela Segura, which identify informal dealers located outside schools and give preventive talks to students.

This, however, seems to be insufficient, since only 8 schools are enrolled in the second project, out of 66 educational units in the city, according to their records.

The situation worries parents who go to see their children every day after school to prevent the teenagers from interacting with the alleged drug dealers, young people who carry backpacks, wear T-shirts, shorts and caps.

With teary eyes and a cracked voice, Nancy C. says that two weeks ago she discovered that her 15-year-old son was using H. "He came to me vomiting, he was cold, but I never thought he would do those things," she says, adding that for now her son does not go to school; she goes on Tuesdays and Thursdays to pick up the homework that is sent home.

Arequipa reports that the sectors with the highest incidence of drug use are the hills of Las Cabras and Redondo, El Recreo, El Arbolito and Colinas del Valle. (Universo, 2015)

JUSTIFICATION

Previous studies such as those previously cited (WHO, Drug Addiction, 2015) (UNODC, 2016) (Universo, 2015) have evidenced the increase in the percentage of drug addiction in the world.

This study aims to analyze the situation of adolescents who suffer from drug addiction, determine what are the predisposing risk factors for this vice, carried out with the help of statistical data obtained at the Hospital Básico Duran, the results will allow us to assess the criteria for which there is drug addiction, and thus seek to reduce the increase that has occurred in recent years and thus raise preventive measures against drug addiction because it is known that this disease affects the whole society and carries a number of clinical complications seriously affecting the health of adolescents. We will seek to promote campaigns that talk about drug addiction by making posters and banners on the subject so that the community in general of the Duran canton is aware of the complications of drug use, especially in adolescents.

It is very important to know the problem of addiction to psychotropic substances because in my training to obtain my degree as a doctor since the first years of undergraduate we have been taught primary health care, to prevent disease and promote health in the community. That is why the study has been conducted to find out what are the causes for an adolescent to fall into this problem, always remembering that they are the future of our country and we must provide all the necessary help.

PROBLEM DETERMINATION

Adolescents from the duran canton during the years 2013 to 2015 presented risk factors for drug addiction with effects for which they attended the HOSPITAL BASICO DURAN and which will be studied in the present rescarch.

The present investigation was carried out:

Nature: it is a basic study of indirect observation, retrospective, cross-sectional and descriptive.

Field Of Research: Public Health.

Location: Hospital Básico Durán

Area: Internal Medicine and Neurology

Period: 2013 to 2015

Aspect: predominant factors

Topic: "Drug addiction and its impact on adolescents in the Durán canton in the years 2013 to 2015 with statistical data from the HOSPITAL BASICO DURAN".

PROBLEM FORMULATION

What are the risk factors for drug addiction in adolescents in duran canton during the period 2013 to 2015?

What are risk factors that determine the choice of drug use?

What complications can occur in adolescents with drug addiction?

What measures should be taken to prevent drug use and abuse that will help us reduce the current rate of drug addiction?

GENERAL AND SPECIFIC OBJECTIVES
GENERAL OBJECTIVE

- To determine which are the risk factors for drug addiction that have an impact on adolescents served in the Duran canton during the years 2013 to 2015.

SPECIFIC OBJECTIVES

- To analyze the risk factors for drug addiction in adolescents.

- To identify the risk factors that expose adolescents between 12 and 16 years of age attending the HOSPITAL BASICO DURAN to the consumption of psychotropic substances.

- Establish action and prevention measures to help eliminate the risk factors for drug addiction among adolescents in the Duran canton.

CHAPTER II

THEORETICAL FRAMEWORK

DEFINITION OF DRUGS

For the WHO, any substance, natural or synthetic, that when consumed can alter the mental and physical activity of people, due to its effects on the Central Nervous System, is a DRUG.

For some authors, such as (Fernandez-Espejo, 2002) a drug is "any natural or synthetic substance that generates addiction, i.e., the imperious or compulsive need to consume again to experience the reward it produces, which is a sensation of pleasure, euphoria, relief of tension, etc".

Thus, the term drug is used to refer to those substances that cause an alteration of the state of mind and are capable of producing addiction. This term includes not only substances that are popularly considered as drugs due to their illegal status, but also various psychotropic drugs and legally consumed substances such as tobacco, alcohol or beverages containing caffeine or theophylline derivatives, such as coffee or tea; as well as substances for domestic or occupational use such as glues, adhesives and volatile solvents.

HISTORY

It can be affirmed that with the appearance of man, the intention to obtain substances capable of producing changes in the state of mind, the level of alertness and the perception of the world also began, and psychoactive substances, more commonly called 'drugs', were discovered and elaborated.

References to the use of stimulant, depressant and hallucinogenic drugs are found in the most ancient writing samples, and it has been observed that in primitive cultures the use of psychoactives almost always had a ritual and magical-religious significance, and the authorities exercised some control over their use through specific laws or through force of habit. (Carvalho, 2007) Technological advances made it possible to learn how to concentrate and isolate the active ingredients of certain drugs. This process began with the alchemists and the distillation of alcohol and reached remarkable efficiency in the 19th century when the alkaloids caffeine, morphine and cocaine were isolated. The invention of the hypodermic syringe allowed for safer forms of administration, which in turn favored the development of new compounds such as heroin, amphetamines and PCP, products of chemical synthesis.

The development of certain drugs provided medicine with powerful elements for the treatment of diseases, the relief of pain and the control of depression; but it also confronted society with an unforeseen phenomenon: the appearance of people who, under the effects of drugs, lost control of their actions, abandoned established norms and committed criminal acts.

The situation was made more dramatic by the fact that users generally came from defined ethnic minorities, who faced even more severe discrimination, with repressive mechanisms based on violence. This is why, in the early stages, drug use was not considered a health problem but rather a social and political issue.

Thus, the last years of the 19th century witnessed important movements that advocated the need to regulate and control the marketing and use of drugs, even going so far as to propose their outright prohibition. However, such initiatives were not new; history already showed important precedents in global efforts to control the abuse of opium and its derivatives.

As a consequence, at the beginning of the twentieth century, campaigns arose that encouraged the proscription of all drugs capable of producing dependence, the so-called 'narcotics' or 'narcotic drugs'. Thus, most countries initially restricted opium, then morphine, cocaine and some synthetic derivatives. (Venum, 2014).

The measures adopted by each country and the international control agreements initially led to a considerable reduction in the number of cases of drug addiction and accidents, but at the same time led to the formation of subway mechanisms dedicated to the production and marketing of illegal drugs, which base their power on violence and their enormous capacity for corruption.

According to (Venum, 2014), In the mid-1960s, a current that questioned the established values was spread throughout the world, posing the search for individual satisfaction beyond conventional activities.

At that time, drug use began to be associated with the search for individual liberation, which led to an explosive increase in consumption worldwide, followed by a notable increase in the actions of drug gangs, widespread violence and crises in international relations as the 'producing' and 'consuming' countries blamed each other for the problem.

However, beyond the international responsibilities and the historical process involved, the concrete fact is that the world today is facing a serious problem, associated with multiple cases of disease and death involving many people and incalculable amounts of money.

The panorama is complicated by the existence of highly dangerous drugs whose use is not only socially accepted but also freely promoted; such is the case of alcohol and tobacco, which fall into the category of social drugs. On the other hand, even today there are ethnic minorities that make ritual and magical-religious use of some drugs as a genuine expression of their respective cultures. (Venum, 2014).

CLASSIFICATION OF DRUGS

Drugs have been classified according to multiple categorization systems, such as the effects they produce on the central nervous system (CONSEP, Drugs, 2012), by their legal status, hard or soft drugs:

The classification of drugs according to the effects they produce at the level of the central nervous system constitutes the most accepted classification system at present. (Yaria, 2015).

Central nervous system depressants or psycholeptics: they inhibit the functioning of the central nervous system, slowing down nervous activity and the rhythm of body functions. Among the effects they produce are relaxation, sedation, drowsiness, sleep, analgesia and even coma. Examples of these substances include alcohol, various types of opiates (heroin, morphine, methadone, etc.), certain psychotropic drugs (such as benzodiazepines or barbiturates), etc.

Stimulants or Psychoanaleptics: produce a general activation of the central nervous system, leading to an increase in bodily functions. A distinction is made between major stimulants (such as cocaine or amphetamines) and minor stimulants (such as nicotine, caffeine, theine, theobromine).

Hallucinogens or Psychodysleptics: also known as disrupters. They produce an altered state of consciousness, distort perception and evoke sensory images without sensory input. Examples of these substances are LSD or synthetic drugs (which, due to the effects they produce, would be considered mixed stimulant-hallucinogenic substances).

According to their legal status, drugs are classified as follows:

Legal drugs: Legal drugs are drugs whose use is not criminalized by t   he   law   . Generally, alcohol, tobacco, coffee and medicines are examples of legal drugs. Even so, there are control mechanisms and, for example, both tobacco and alcohol are subject to special taxes, normally much higher than normal taxes, and their sale is controlled. Another example is that of some medicines, which can only be purchased under the prescription of a licensed physician.

Illegal drugs: Illegal drugs are those drugs whose use is prohibited or penalized by law. For example: cocaine, heroin, and those drugs that have been proven to be harmful.

Hard drugs and soft drugs:

The difference between a hard drug and a soft drug is that hard drugs cause addiction and/or a physical and psychological dependence, while a soft drug only causes a single addiction and/or dependence, which can be on a psychological level only or on a physical level only.

Originally, this distinction was intended to distinguish highly addictive drugs that cause serious damage to health (hard drugs) from those that are not very addictive, which do not present a serious risk to the user (soft drugs). (Claudio, 2014)

CONCEPTUAL FRAMEWORK

ADDICTION

According to the World Health Organization (WHO) it is a physical and psychoemotional disease that creates a dependence or need for a substance, activity or relationship. It is characterized by a set of signs and symptoms, involving biological, genetic, psychological and social factors.

It is a progressive and fatal disease, characterized by continuous episodes of uncontrolled, distorted thinking and denial of the disease. (WHO, Addictions, 2016).

DRUG ADDICTION

Drug addiction is a disorder characterized by an uncontrollable desire to consume a certain substance. It is a disease that originates in the brain of a large number of human beings, the disease is characterized by its chronicity or long duration, its progressiveness and relapses. The abuse of any type of drugs for purposes other than the initial ones prescribed, when the prescription exists. (WHO, Glossary of terms, 2008).

TOLERANCE

When the drug has caused certain physiological alterations in the organism, the phenomenon of tolerance appears, which means that the individual requires increasingly higher doses to achieve effects of the same intensity as it was initially, i.e. the organism has developed tolerance with the consequent risk of contracting chronic intoxication.

It can occur rapidly and the degree of it depends on each type of drug. (WHO, Glossary of Terms, 2008)

PHARMACODEPENDENCE

According to the World Health Organization (WHO), drug dependence is the psychological and physical state caused by the reciprocal action between a living organism and a drug, characterized by behavioral changes and other reactions that always involve an irrepressible impulse to take the drug periodically or continuously in order to experience its psychological and sometimes physical effects to avoid the discomfort produced by deprivation. Some drugs have harmful effects on the body and generate a high tolerance relatively quickly, this has led many people including young people and children to self-medicate. (PHARMACODEPENDENCIES, 2015).

MEDICATIONS

The National Council on Narcotic Drugs and Psychotropic Substances (CONSEP) defines drugs as all preparations or pharmaceutical forms used for therapeutic purposes for the cure or prevention of diseases in humans or animals. Nowadays, drug addicts are not only those who consume marijuana, heroin, cocaine or other illicit substances, since the ingestion of certain drugs that are easily available, such as tranquilizers and amphetamines, are capable of generating an addiction and, consequently, they can become drug addicts. (CONSEP, Perceptions on drug use, 2015) This results in some cases in physical dependence, i.e. a state of biological adaptation manifested by more or less intense physiological disorders when the drug is abruptly discontinued, and psychological dependence which means the compulsive use of a drug without the development of physical dependence, to procure a pleasure or to dissipate a state of discomfort. (Technical Secretariat for Drugs, 2016).

RISK AND PROTECTIVE FACTORS FOR DRUG USE.

One of the most widely accepted theories in the field of drug use prevention is that of protective and risk factors. Factors or conditions that are associated with a low probability of occurrence of risk behavior, in this case drug use, are called protective factors. In contrast, factors or conditions that increase the probability of initiating or maintaining drug use are called risk factors.

THE FAMILY

Since the family is the nucleus of any society, it is currently affected by this social problem, so it is important that we emphasize its importance:

FAMILY STRUCTURE AND COMPOSITION

Many studies have pointed out that both the absence of a parent from the family and the fact that one of the parents remarries could be conceptualized as risk factors that predict future drug use by children.

FAMILY DISCIPLINE

The variable parental control or monitoring has been associated with the etiology of drug abuse in adolescence. Factors such as the absence of maternal involvement, the absence or inconsistency of parental discipline and low parental aspirations for their children's education were found to predict their initiation of drug use. (Andrews, 1987).

AFFECTIVE RELATIONSHIPS AND COMMUNICATION   ,
AFFECTION/PARENTAL-FILIAL BONDING

Most studies agree that parent-child interactions characterized by a lack of connection and maternal over-involvement in activities with children appear to be related to young adolescents' initiation of drug use. Conversely, positive family relationships based on deep parent-child bonding correlate with a lower likelihood of youth exhibiting behavioral problems and initiation into substance use.

FAMILY COMMUNICATION

Many studies generally confirm the importance of parental-child communication but, with reference to the specific problem of drugs, argue that although the relationship with parents has a special role in the life of the young person, the one established with friends can be much more relevant.

FAMILY COHESION

It is argued that, with respect to drug use, the probability that young people manifest such behavior decreases as their participation in family decisions increases and, on the contrary, increases as the degree of disagreement in the family increases.

FAMILY CONFLICT

Generically, it is argued that raising children in high-conflict families is an important risk factor for both the development of behavioral disorders in general and for substance use.

FAMILY ATTITUDES AND BEHAVIORS TOWARDS DRUG USE

Parental drug use has been repeatedly associated with adolescent initiation of intoxicant use and with frequency of drug use. In this case, this positive correlation has been found for most legal and illegal drugs. Regarding the more attitudinal factor of parental modeling, it is important to note that parental permissive attitudes towards substance use are perceived by young people as being of equal or greater importance than actual parental use (Muñoz, 2001).

PROTECTIVE FACTORS

There are many factors that currently act as a protective barrier to prevent children and adolescents from consuming any type of psychotropic substances, which are mentioned below according to the levels at which they occur:

PERSONNEL LEVEL

Among the protective factors at the personal level are: the capacity for autonomy, independence, empathy, satisfaction with what has been received, tendency to approach people and situations at the intellectual level, positive self-esteem, assertive attitudes, existence of a life project, development of healthy activities (membership in youth clubs, music, painting), and physical exercise.

COMMUNAL AND SOCIAL LEVEL, PROTECTION FACTORS

Among the protective factors at the community and social level, the microenvironments where the person develops are taken into account, such as: school, college, university, workplaces, recreational places, the street, among others, as long as they favor the integral formation of the person.one of the groups of risk factors that have attracted most attention among researchers has been family factors. Drug use is based on a socialization process in which the family influences as a transmitter of beliefs, values and habits that later condition the probability of drug use.

LEGAL FRAMEWORK

Comprehensive prevention of drug use and abuse among children should be based on a thorough understanding of the social and economic environment of Ecuadorian families and children, factors that contribute to its origin. The vision of the general characteristics of the reality of Ecuadorian children and adolescents and the actions of the State in its different aspects, has identified new challenges to which it is necessary to respond and that make it necessary to reorient efforts and establish lines of action with the purpose of elaborating a comprehensive prevention proposal that seeks an effective coordination of the various sectors and institutions.

The following is the legal framework on which our research work is based:

LAW ON NARCOTIC AND PSYCHOTROPIC SUBSTANCES

Art. 1.- Objective.- The objective of this Law is to combat and eradicate the production, supply, improper use and illicit trafficking of narcotic and psychotropic substances, in order to protect the community from the dangers arising from these activities.

Article 2 - Declaration of national interest - The attainment of the objective determined in this Law, the actions carried out for its application and, in particular, the plans, programs and activities adopted or executed by the competent agencies shall be declared of national interest. The institutions, agencies and servants of the public sector and the natural or juridical persons of the private sector are obliged to provide the information and to render the collaboration determined by this Law or established by the authorities in charge of its application.

TITLE TWO PREVENTION

Art. 19.- Preventive activities: The public institutions and agencies, in application of the plans and programs for the prevention of the abuse of controlled substances, shall develop, in the areas of their competence or activity, under the supervision of the Executive Secretariat and in coordination and collaboration with the entities and persons they deem appropriate, the campaigns tending to achieve the objectives of this Law.

Art. 20.- Preventive education: The programs of all levels and modalities of the national education system shall include pedagogical approaches and methodologies that develop the formation of an individual personality and a social conscience oriented to the prevention of the abuse of controlled substances.

The authorities of the national education system and the directors of public, municipal and private educational establishments and teachers in general should actively participate in prevention campaigns.

TITLE THREE

Art. 29.- Abuse of controlled substances: Abuse of controlled substances is understood to be any use that is not therapeutic.

Article 30 - Compulsory examination and treatment - Members of the security forces are obliged to immediately take any person who appears to be under the harmful effects of a controlled substance to a psychiatric hospital or assistance center, so that the physicians of the corresponding health center may verify whether he is under the effect of such substances. If so, they will evaluate if there is intoxication and the degree it has reached. If this is the case, they will immediately order the appropriate treatment. The treatment to be carried out in special centers shall be performed in those previously qualified and authorized by the Executive Secretariat, in coordination with the Ministry of Public Health (Law 108, 1990).

The state guarantees through this law that the CONSEP is in charge of drug control and eradication. The CONSEP must watch over and provide economic resources for the realization of educational projects or at least promote them for the prevention of drug use in educational institutions. In addition to providing rehabilitation services to young people who have entered the world of drugs.

SUBSTANCE USE ASSOCIATED WITH PSYCHIATRIC PATHOLOGIES

When we talk about drug addiction, we must be clear that it is itself classified as a mental illness, since it interrupts and alters the normal categorization of needs and desires, replacing them with new priorities linked to the acquisition and consumption of psychotropic drugs. Compulsive behaviors impair the ability to control impulses, leading to a progressive degradation in the interaction with the environment. This picture corresponds to a common symptomatology in psychopathologies.

A large number of drug addicts are also diagnosed with other mental illnesses, and vice versa. Without going any further, drug addicts are twice as likely to suffer from pathologies associated with mood or anxiety, which also occurs in the opposite direction.

But why is there such a marked comorbidity between drug dependence and mental disorder? Although drug addiction disorders occur concurrently with other psychopathologies, this does not mean that one causes the other, although one may appear earlier and the other later. Indeed, it is often complex to dictate which of the disorders emerged first and why. However, studies indicate the following points as reasons why it is common for these illnesses to present comorbidly:

- **Drug dependence often causes the symptoms of other psychopathology.** For example, some cannabis smokers with certain underlying vulnerabilities may be at increased risk of developing psychotic conditions.
- **Mental illness can lead to drug use**, probably as a form of self-medication. People suffering from anxiety or depression are more likely to use alcohol, smoking or other drugs or psychotropic drugs that may temporarily alleviate their symptoms.

These psychopathologies can also be explained by shared risk factors, such as:

- **The addition of genetic vulnerabilities.** Some genetic predispositions may increase susceptibility to both drug addiction and other psychopathology, or may have an increased risk for the second pathology once the first has appeared.
- **The addition of risk factors in the environment.** Stress, substance abuse at a young age or childhood trauma can lead to drug addiction, which in turn can lead to other mental disorders.
- **Activation of similar brain areas.** For example, brain systems that are activated during gratification or stress are altered by substance use and may be abnormal in people with certain psychopathologies.
- **Substance abuse pathologies and other mental disorders are developmental disorders.** They usually appear during adolescence or even during puberty, just at the periods when the brain and nervous system undergo abrupt changes due to their development. The consumption of drugs at this stage of life can modify the brain structures in such a way that the risk of suffering from psychopathologies will be greater in the future. Thus, when there is an early symptomatology of mental illness it is usually linked to a higher risk of drug addiction in the future.

Studies carried out in the Community of Madrid between 2006 and 2008 indicated that the concurrence of drug dependence disorders with mental illness occurred mainly in men (80%), with an average age of up to 37 years, single (58%) with primary school education (46%).

The most common mental illnesses in these individuals are personality disorders, suicide risk, hypomanic episodes, anxiety disorders and major depression.

Two or more substances were used by 55% of the subjects evaluated. Cocaine (63%), alcohol (61%) and cannabis (23%) were the most reported drugs.

AUTHOR'S OPINION

The purpose of my study is to determine the predisposing causes of drug addiction in adolescents. To analyze the results of the review of the clinical histories of the patients attended at the HOPSPITAL BASICO DURAN and to reach a conclusion as to the pathologies for which the patients were admitted or attended by the INTERNAL MEDICINE service.

HYPOTHESIS

Through the study of the medical records of adolescent patients who are substance abusers, the incidence of these cases and the psychopathologies associated with this clinical picture in patients treated in the emergency and n the hospitalization area of the HOSPITAL BASICO DURAN during the years 2013-2015 will be obtained.

RESEARCH VARIABLES
INDEPENDENT VARIABLE

Adolescent drug addicts.

DEPENDENT VARIABLE

Age Sex

Type of drug consumed Time of drug use

CHAPTER III

MATERIALS AND METHODS

CHARACTERIZATION OF THE WORK AREA (NATIONAL, ZONAL, PROVINCIAL, CANTONAL AND LOCAL)

Ecuador, zonal 8, Guayas, Guayaquil, Hospital Básico Durán.

PERIOD OF INVESTIGATION

The period of this research is from the year 2013 to 2015 according to the cases reported according to the statistics department of the Hospital Básico Durán on drug addiction.

TYPE OF RESEARCH

According to the characteristics and nature of this cross-sectional, retrospective, non-experimental observational and descriptive research, since it is based on a certain reality that is happening at the Hospital Básico Durán. Data was collected on the incidence, risk factors, causes and complications associated with drug addiction in adolescents, the source of information being books, encyclopedias, medical articles, magazines and updated web pages.

UNIVERSE AND SAMPLE

UNIVERSE: All patients with a diagnosis of drug addiction ambulatory or hospitalized, treated in the Internal Medicine area in the period from 2013 to 2015 at the Hospital Básico Durán.

SAMPLE: All adolescent patients (12-16 years old) with a diagnosis of drug addiction treated in the Internal Medicine area from 2013 to 2015 at the Hospital Básico Durán.

FEASIBILITY

This study was carried out on the basis of statistical data provided by the statistics department of the hospital where the study was carried out, with the prior authorization of the institution's Director of Teaching.

25

INCLUSION AND EXCLUSION CRITERIA
Inclusion criteria:

- All patients admitted to the emergency department of the HOSPITAL BASICO DURAN during the period 2013-2015.
- Any patient who is seen with a diagnosis of substance use between the ages of 12 and 16 years old.
- Any patient who has associated with substance use psychopathologies such as delirium, dementia, anxiety disorders, bipolar disorders, conduct disorder, personality disorders, psychotic disorders, depression.

Exclusion criteria:

- Patients admitted without a diagnosis of substance use.
- Patients admitted with a diagnosis of substance use who do not fall within the established age range.
- Patients who have been admitted in a period of time different from that established.

DEVELOPMENT OF VARIABLES.

VARIABLES INDEPENDENT	DEFINITION	INDICATORS	RATING SCALE	SOURCE
DRUG ADDICTION	It is the dependence on substances that affect the central nervous system and brain functions, producing alterations in behavior. behavior, perception, judgment and emotions.	TYPES OF DRUGS	MARIHUANA COCAINE HACHE CRACK HEROIN LSD MORPHINE, BENZODIAZEPINES	MEDICAL HISTORY

VARIABLE DEPENDENT	DEFINITION	INDICATORS	RATING SCALE	SOURCE
TEENAGE DRUG ADDICTS		AGE	12+18	MEDICAL HISTORY
		SEX	MALE AND FEMALE	
		TYPE OF DRUG CONSUMED	COCAINE MARIJUANA, ACHE	
		TIME OF DRUG ADDICTION	MONTHS, 1 YEAR, > than 2 years	

OPERATIONALIZATION OF RESEARCH INSTRUMENTS
Medical records.

The present research study was based on the review of the medical records of each patient stored in a computerized system called AS-400 with prior notice to the authorities of the HOSPITAL BASICO DURAN and with the help of the Statistics Department, which provided me with the same in order to properly order the information on the patients who used substances and the associated psychopathologies.

Bibliographic sheets

The literary resources of several authors collected in books, articles, magazines and other documents that contributed to the development of this research were used for this investigation.

TYPE OF RESEARCH

The present study was descriptive, retrospective, conducted by indirect observation of medical records collected in the period 2013 - 2015, which were compiled by means of a filter chosen by means of the ICD-10 disease coding system.

PROJECT IMPLEMENTATION SCHEDULE (2016-2017)

ACTIVITIES	Aug.	Sept	Oct	Nov	Dec	Jan	Feb	Sea	Apr	May
Meeting with the Thesis Tutor	▓									
Approach to Project		▓								
Elaboration of the Chapter I		▓								
Elaboration of the Chapter II		▓								
Elaboration of the Chapter III			▓							
Approval of the Project of the Preliminary project				▓						
Review Bibliographic					▓					

Collection of Data						■				
Execution of the work of Qualification							■			
Structuring of the Research Design							■			
Elaboration of the Chapter IV							■			
Elaboration of the Chapter V								■		
Elaboration of the Chapter VI									■	
Presentation of the Degree Work										■

BIOETHICAL CONSIDERATIONS

According to the clinical practice guidelines for the management of adolescent substance users, patients with signs of acute intoxication, psychotropic substance dependence syndrome and withdrawal syndrome identified can be stabilized and sent home to continue their outpatient control through a program managed by the Hospital Básico Duran in charge of the Internal Medicine Department, comprising Dr. María Eugenia Yépez and other collaborators, in which the patients as well as the families of the adolescents involved are committed to rigorous control in order to combat this disease. Therefore, the main objective is to identify the presence of indicators with warning signs:

- Patients who become complicated in the therapeutic process.
- Patients with multiple relapses within the therapeutic process.
- Patients with psychiatric comorbidity. (e.g. psychosis)
- Patients with unmanageable medical comorbidity at this level (e.g. liver cirrhosis).
- Patient with detected addictive symptoms.

HUMAN AND PHYSICAL RESOURCES
Humans

- Collaboration of the Statistics Department upon request addressed to the Medical Direction of the HOSPITAL BASICO DURAN.
- Researcher (Medical Intern)
- Degree work tutor

Institutional

- DURAN BASIC HOSPITAL
- Faculty of Medical Sciences
- University of Guayaquil.

Physicists

- Furniture, Materials and supplies, Stationery, Books, Office supplies, Photocopies.
- Computer, Printer, Pendrive
- Books, Articles, Journals, Medical Records (AS-400).
- Vehicular transportation (own vehicle)

Financial

The expenses generated in the research that were fully paid by the researcher (Medical Intern).

METHODOLOGY FOR THE ANALYSIS OF RESULTS

The results were tabulated by means of the Excel computer program, where the tables and percentages of each variable were obtained. In addition, statistical bar graphs were elaborated to proceed to their respective analysis and interpretation and to be able to issue the respective conclusions and recommendations.

CHAPTER IV RESULTS AND DISCUSSION

ANALYSIS AND INTERPRETATION

Distribution of age and gender in the incidence of cases of substance use in adolescents seen in the emergency department of the HOSPITAL BASICO DURAN during the period 2013-2015.

TABLE 1.

GENRE	Male		Female		Total	
AGES	#	%	#	%	#	%
12 - 16 years old		32%		9%		41%
16- 18 years		39.6 6%	58	19. 34 %		59%
TOTAL	2 1 5	71.6 6%		28. 34 %		100%

Source: Department of Statistics of the HOSPITAL BASICO DURAN

Prepared by: Katerine J. Sacoto Quinteros

FIGURE 1

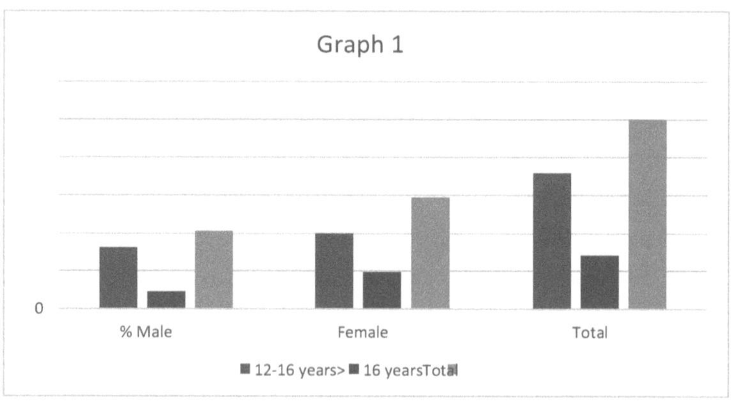

Source: Department of Statistics of the HOSPITAL BASICO DURAN

Prepared by: Katerine J. Sacoto Quinteros

The results of the clinical records of cases of adolescents related to drug use attended at the Hospital Básico Duran during the period 2013- 2015 showed that 71.66 % occurred in the male gender in relation to the female gender that presented a lower value of 28.34%, where 41% occurred in the age between 12 to 16 years and 59% in age from 16 to 18 years.

Prevalence of gender in patients with drug use-related problems.

TABLE 2.

Genre	Frequency	Percentage
Male		78.05
Female		21.95
Total		

Source: Department of Statistics of the HOSPITAL BASICO DURAN

Prepared by: Katerine J. Sacoto Quinteros

FIGURE 2

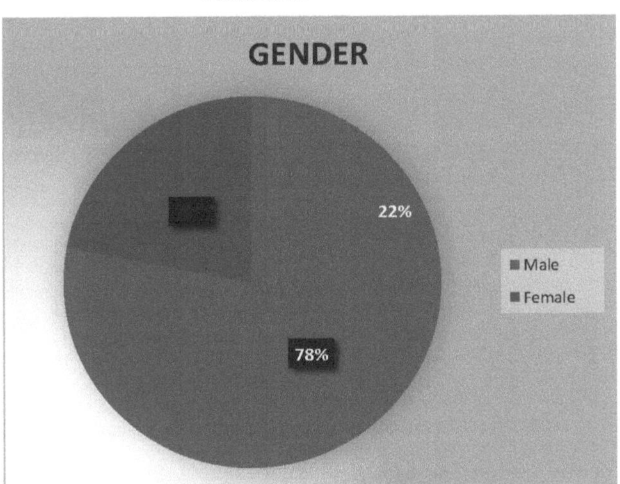

Source: Department of Statistics of the HOSPITAL BASICO DURAN

Prepared by: Katerine J. Sacoto Quinteros

According to the verification of the medical records, it was determined that 78% of the cases of adolescent substance users at the Neurosciences Institute of the Junta de Beneficencia de Guayaquil were male and 22% were female and belonged to a population living in the marginal urban sector of the Duran canton, adolescents of limited resources and with a tendency to consume low-cost substances (hashish).

Type of drug in the incidence of substance use cases in adolescents attended in the emergency and outpatient departments of the HOSPITAL BASICO DURAN during the years 2013-2015.

TABLE 3.

Type of drug	Frequency	Percentage
HACHE		30.90
Marijuana		9.75
Hallucinogens - LSD	5	4.06
Cocaine		2.44
Volatile solvents		14.64
Multiple drugs		38.21
Total		100,00

Source: Department of Statistics of the HOSPITAL BASICO DURAN

Prepared by: Katerine J. Sacoto Quinteros

FIGURE 3

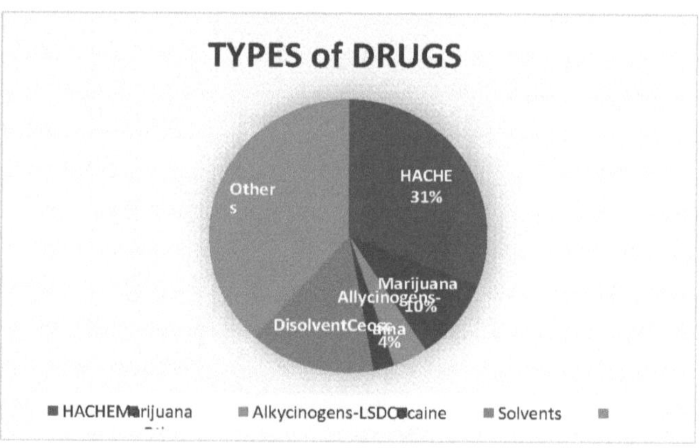

Source: Department of Statistics of the HOSPITAL BASICO DURAN

Prepared by: Katerine J. Sacoto Quinteros

The results of the clinical histories collected during the years 2013-2015, where the cases of adolescent substance-consuming patients in the canton Duran and attended at the HOSPITAL BASICO DURAN were recorded, showed that the most used and consumed drug because of its low cost and easy accessibility is the ``hache" a mega derivative of cocaine with a percentage of consumption of 31% followed by solvents with 15%, marijuana at 10%, hallucinogens and cocaine in low percentages 4% and 2% respectively.

Onset and frequency of psychotropic substance use in adolescents seen in the emergency and outpatient departments of the HOSPITAL BASICO DURAN during the years 2013-2015.

TABLE 4.

FREQUENCY OF CONSUMPTION	1 - 2 TIMES A WEEK		MASDE 3 THE WEEK		TOTAL	
HOME OF CONSUMPTION	F	%	F	%	F	%
10 years	1	0.81		2.44		3.25
11 years	1	0.81		1.63		2.44
12 years		4.88		9.75		14.63
13 years		12.20		11.38		23.58
14 years		13.01		12.19		25.20
15 years		11.39		6.50		17.89
16 years old	5	4.05		8.95		
TOTAL	58	47.15		52.85		

Source: Department of Statistics of the HOSPITAL BASICO DURAN
Prepared by: Katerine J. Sacoto Quinteros

The clinical histories of the patients where the cases of adolescent substance users in the canton of Duran and treated at the HOSPITAL BASICO DURAN were recorded, showed that the start of substance use occurs most frequently with 25.20% at 14 years of age and the highest frequency of use that occurs 1 to 2 times a week is 13.01% in adolescents 14 years of age and more than 3 times a week is 12.19% in adolescents 14 and 15 years of age.

Reason for consultation in the incidence of cases of substance use in adolescents seen in the emergency and outpatient departments of the HOSPITAL BASICO DURAN during the years 2013-2015.

TABLE 6.

Reason for inquiry	Frequency	Percentage
Acute Intoxication	58	47.15
Syndrome dependence		26.02
Syndrome Abstinence		26.83
Total		

Source: Department of Statistics of the HOSPITAL BASICO DURAN

Prepared by: Katerine J. Sacoto Quinteros

The reports of the clinical histories collected from the period 2013-2015 treated at the Hospital Básico Duran, reflected as the most common cause of reason for consultation with 47.15% cases of acute intoxication in which increased sensitivity to external stimuli, alteration in the perception of objects, slowing in the appreciation of the passage of time, anxiety, etc. are observed.In 26.83% there is a withdrawal syndrome that generally presents with dyspnea, palpitations, anger, aggressiveness, decreased appetite or weight loss, anxiety, restlessness, insomnia, chills, depression, epigastric pain, tremors and sweating, etc.; and in 26.02% there is a dependence syndrome characterized by anxiety, mood swings, unmotivated laughter or crying, myalgia, arthralgia, etc.;

DISCUSSION

Substance use in adolescents is a serious public health problem and there is little attention and few resources for its prevention and treatment, but more disturbing is the high percentage of consumption of these substances in our young Ecuadorians and this as a small sample in the canton of Duran. Regarding the data obtained in the present study, there was a predominance of 78% in the male gender in relation to the female gender which presented the lowest value with 22%; where 41% occurred between the ages of 12 to 16 years and 59% occurred between the ages of 16 to 18 years.

According to this study, the drug most consumed by adolescents is hashish (31%) due to its ease of purchase and low price; its age of onset was 25.20% at 14 years of age and the frequency of consumption of 1 to 2 times a week was 13.01% in adolescents of 14 years of age, and consumption more than 3 times a week was 12.19% in adolescents of 14 years of age.

The most frequent reason for consultation in the emergency department was acute intoxication (47.15%), withdrawal syndrome (26.83%) and dependence syndrome (26.02%).

CHAPTER V

CONCLUSIONS

Regarding the data obtained in the present study, there was a predominance of the male sex in relation to the female sex and the highest number of cases occurred between the ages of 13 and 15 years.

It was determined that the drug most consumed by adolescents is hashish because of its easy accessibility and low cost, the age of onset of consumption was frequently at 14 years of age and the majority of the population consumes drugs more than 3 times a week.

The most frequent reason for consultation in the emergency department was acute intoxication, followed by withdrawal syndrome and finally by dependence syndrome characterized by anxiety, mood swings, unmotivated laughter or crying, myalgia and arthralgia.

CHAPTER VI

RECOMMENDATIONS OR PROPOSALS

- Strengthen continuing education plans for medical personnel for the timely identification of signs of acute substance intoxication in order to prevent fatal cases of the disease.

- Provide information to family members about prevention measures and treatment plans for adolescents who wish to stop using.

- Seek medical and psychological care in a timely manner.

- Provide talks on the subject at strategic locations within the Hospital.

- The data obtained in this study could bring us closer to a more accurate and rapid prevention scheme to avoid the complications of substance use, starting with the appropriate management when the warning signs are just beginning to appear.

BIBLIOGRAPHY

- Andrews, K. and. (1987). Drugs risk factors. England.

- Carvalho, J. T. (2007). HISTORY OF DRUGS AND THE WAR OF THEIR DIFFUSION. Legal News, 2-4.

- Claudio, P. (2014). DRUGS, TYPES,CLASSIFICATION,ADDICTION, DEFINITION, CONCEPTS. HEALTH and MEDICINE, 2-6.

- CONSEP. (2012). Drugs. Drugs.

- CONSEP. (2015). Perceptions about drug use. Relatos de Docentes de enseñanza media en la ciudad de Quito.

- DRUG DEPENDENCE. (2015). Pharmacodependence. In FARMACODEPENDENCIAS, Farmacodependencia un enfoque disciplinario (p. 113). Mexico: Direccion genreal de prevencion del delito y servicios a la comunidad de la Re3publica and UNICEF.

- Fernandez-Espejo. (2002). Neurobiological basis of drug addiction. Revista de Neurologia, 659-664.

- WHO. (2008). Glossary of Terms. World Health Organization, 61.

- WHO. (2008). Glossary of terms. World Health Organization, 52.

- WHO. (2015). Drug addiction.

- WHO. (2016). Addictions. DRUGS.

- Technical Secretariat on Drugs. (2016). Prevencion de Drogas. Retrieved from http://www.prevenciondrogas.gob.ec/

- Universo, E. (August 16, 2015). Drug dealing worries Durán. El Universo, p. 5.

- UNODC. (2016). WORLD DRUG REPORT. NEW YORK.

- Venum. (2014). Drug Problems. PERU: pag. 15.

- Yaria, J. A. (2015). GUIA BASICA DE ADICCIONES. MEXICO.

- Andrews, K. and. (1987). Drugs risk factors. England.

- Carvalho, J. T. (2007). HISTORY OF DRUGS AND THE WAR OF THEIR DIFFUSION. Legal News, 2-4.

- Claudio, P. (2014). DRUGS, TYPES,CLASSIFICATION,ADDICTION, DEFINITION, CONCEPTS. HEALTH and MEDICINE, 2-6.

- CONSEP. (2012). Drugs. Drugs.

- CONSEP. (2015). Perceptions about drug use. Relatos de Docentes de enseñanza media en la ciudad de Quito.

- DRUG DEPENDENCE. (2015). Pharmacodependence. In FARMACODEPENDENCIAS, Farmacodependencia un enfoque disciplinario (p. 113). Mexico: Direccion genreal de prevencion del delito y servicios a la comunidad de la Re3publica and UNICEF.

- Fernandez-Espejo. (2002). Neurobiological basis of drug addiction. Revista de Neurologia, 659-664.

- WHO. (2008). Glossary of Terms. World Health Organization, 61.

- WHO. (2008). Glossary of terms. World Health Organization, 52.

- WHO. (2015). Drug addiction.

- WHO. (2016). Addictions. DRUGS.

- Technical Secretariat on Drugs. (2016). Prevencion de Drogas. Retrieved from http://www.prevenciondrogas.gob.ec/

- Universo, E. (August 16, 2015). Drug dealing worries Durán. El Universo, p. 5.

- UNODC. (2016). WORLD DRUG REPORT. NEW YORK.

- Venum. (2014). Drug Problems. PERU: pag. 15.

- Yaria, J. A. (2015). GUIA BASICA DE ADICCIONES. MEXICO.

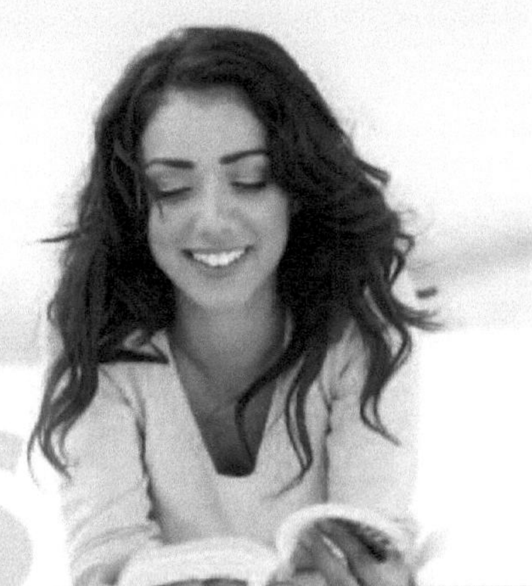

Buy your books fast and straightforward online - at one of world's fastest growing online book stores! Environmentally sound due to Print-on-Demand technologies.

Buy your books online at
www.morebooks.shop

Kaufen Sie Ihre Bücher schnell und unkompliziert online – auf einer der am schnellsten wachsenden Buchhandelsplattformen weltweit! Dank Print-On-Demand umwelt- und ressourcenschonend produziert.

Bücher schneller online kaufen
www.morebooks.shop

KS OmniScriptum Publishing
Brivibas gatve 197
LV-1039 Riga, Latvia
Telefax: +371 686 204 55

info@omniscriptum.com
www.omniscriptum.com

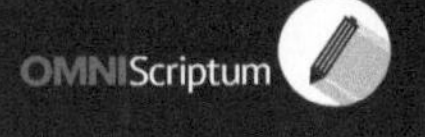

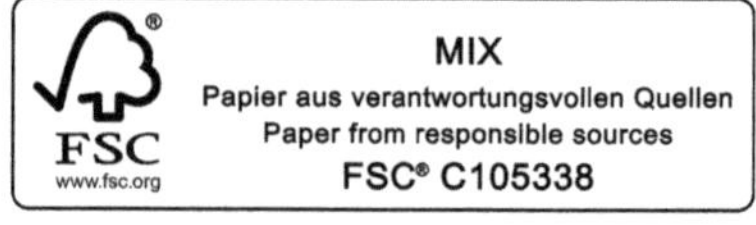

Printed by Books on Demand GmbH, Norderstedt / Germany